Pocket Picture Guides

Skin Signs of Systemic Disease

An **Essential Slide Collection of Skin Signs of Systemic Disease,** based on the material in this book, is available. The collection consists of numbered 35mm colour transparencies of each illustration in the book, and each section is accompanied by a slide index for easy reference. The material is presented in an attractive binder, which also contains a copy of the Pocket Picture Guide. The Essential Slide Collection is available from:

Gower Medical Publishing

Middlesex House,
34–42 Cleveland Street,
London W1P 5FB, UK.

101 5th Avenue,
New York, NY. 10003,
USA.

Pocket Picture Guides

Skin Signs of Systemic Disease

Denis E. Sharvill FRCP

Formerly Consultant Dermatologist
SE Kent, Canterbury and Thanet
Health District, UK

J.B. Lippincott Company • Philadelphia
Gower Medical Publishing • London • New York

Distributed in all countries except the USA & Canada by:
Harper & Row International,
10 East 53rd Street,
New York, NY. 10022, USA.

Distributed in the USA & Canada by:
J.B. Lippincott Company,
East Washington Square,
Philadelphia, PA. 19105, USA.

Library of Congress Catalog Number: 87-82133

British Library Cataloguing in Publication Data

Sharvill, Denis E.
    Skin Signs of Systemic Disease.
    1. Man. Systemic diseases. Symptoms: Skin disorders
    I. Title II. Series
    616.072

ISBN: 0-397-44574-1 (Lippincott/Gower)

Project Editor: Michele Campbell
Design: Chris Inns

Printed in Hong Kong by Imago Publishing Ltd.
Set in Sabon and Frutiger by Dawkins Typesetters, London.

PREFACE

In this book a range of conditions are illustrated which, although not seen every day, are certainly not rare. They are important not only because they may indicate serious underlying illness, such as malignancy or a metabolic disorder, but also because they are striking conditions in their own right, which require proper diagnosis and, where possible, appropriate treatment. While some of these conditions can be grouped together under a general heading such as 'collagen disease' or 'lymphoma', others cannot be put into any simple classification, so that many apparently randomly selected and unrelated conditions will be illustrated within the same section.

All photographs, except Fig. 105, were taken by the author on Kodachrome film. Fig. 105 was provided by the Department of Pathology, Kent and Canterbury Hospital.

D. E. S. London

A more general pictorial account of dermatology is available in 'Skin Diseases' also by D.E. Sharvill, published in the first series of Pocket Picture Guides.

CONTENTS

CUTANEOUS MANIFESTATIONS OF SYSTEMIC DISEASE

Autoimmune and Collagen Diseases

This section covers a group of related diseases which are problematical in every respect, causing difficulties in diagnosis, classification and treatment, even for the specialist. In some cases they overlap and are difficult to distinguish when they present to the dermatologist, the general physician or, increasingly these days, to the immunologist.

These diseases were previously grouped together under the title of collagen diseases, which was never very satisfactory. They cannot all be called autoimmune diseases either, although in most cases there are circulating antibodies, or antibodies in the skin, or both.

Lupus erythematosus

Although in Britain physicians and rheumatologists regard systemic lupus erythematosus as a relatively common disease, a fully developed dermatological presentation is rare. Very commonly however, patients suffering from conditions such as rosacea, photodermatitis, angio-oedema, contact dermatitis or even recurrent erysipelas are referred to skin clinics with the diagnosis of systemic lupus erythematosus.

Discoid lupus erythematosus, which dermatologists see quite often, is in most respects a different disease, although there are borderline cases in which it is difficult to make a precise diagnosis. This occurs when, in addition to the typical skin changes of discoid lupus erythematosus, one or two immunological or haematological abnormalities are present to suggest systemic lupus erythematosus. Occasionally, cases of discoid lupus erythematosus are transformed into systemic lupus erythematosus, but this is not common.

It is perhaps worth mentioning here that abbreviations must be used with care because their use varies with time and geographical location. DLE, for example, may currently be used as an abbreviation for discoid lupus erythematosus, but it was previously held to mean disseminated lupus erythematosus, now called SLE.

Systemic lupus erythematosus (SLE)

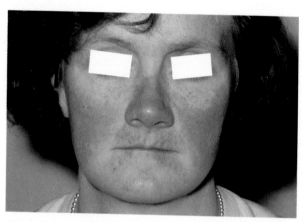

Fig. 1 A bat's-wing erythema on the face. This is widely recognized as characteristic of SLE, but is a rare presentation of the disease in Britain. It is usually seen in young women who present with pyrexia and malaise and until steroids were introduced, the prognosis for such cases was very poor. After 10 days of systemic steroids the erythema on the face and arms had disappeared. It was previously thought that SLE of this type was an absolute indication for steroid therapy, but this is no longer necessarily so. Many such patients will improve quite satisfactorily with bed-rest or antimalarial drugs.

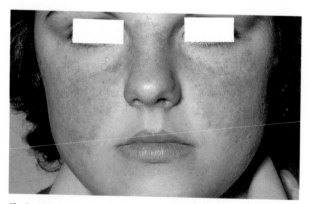

Fig. 2 This child with systemic lupus erythematosus shows facial mooning. The latter is a side-effect of steroid treatment for severe renal involvement. It is interesting to note that in this case a small dose of steroids controlled the kidneys but not the skin.

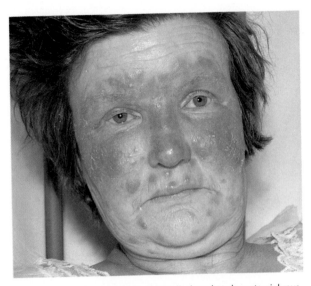

Fig. 3 A spectacular rash which was initially thought to be systemic lupus erythematosus. During one week in hospital, however, it disappeared completely without any active treatment and was probably intense erythema multiforme. The condition did not recur.

Discoid lupus erythematosus (DLE)

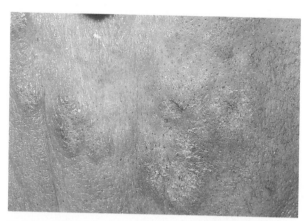

Fig. 4 Typical discoid lupus erythematosus on the face with telangiectasia, atrophy and plugging of the hair follicles. If the scales are carefully lifted off with forceps, the horny plug from the follicular orifice can be seen with a hand lens.

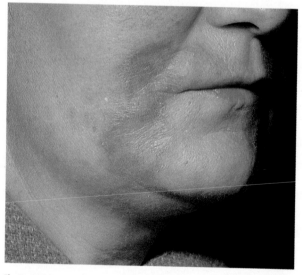

Fig. 5 This is a purely erythematous lesion of discoid lupus erythematosus on the chin.

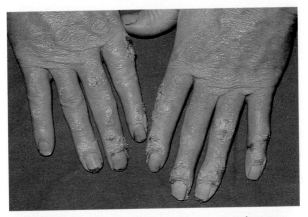

Fig. 6 The hyperkeratotic type of lupus erythematosus may be seen on the hands.

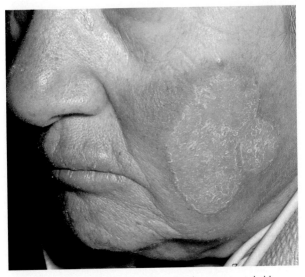

Fig. 7 This is an intermediate type of lupus erythematosus, probably caused by mysoline, presenting like discoid lupus erythematosus but with systemic changes. These changes were not, however, typical of SLE.

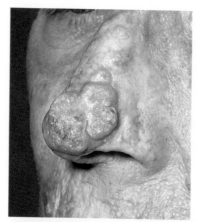

Fig. 8 An inactive and 'burnt out' case of discoid lupus erythematosus of many years standing, with disfiguring hypertrophic lesions on the nose. The lesions were shaved off at skin level and the bases cauterized under local anaesthetic. The cosmetic result was perfect.

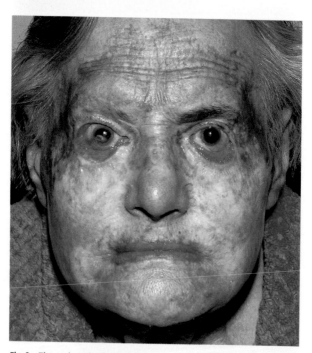

Fig. 9 The end result of severe discoid lupus erythematosus, which was intermittently active for over 50 years. It was originally treated with galvanocautery, tincture of perchloride of iron and carbon dioxide snow. This resulted in gross scarring, ectropion and corneal damage.

Scleroderma

This word is used as a section heading, not as a diagnosis, to include many conditions characterized by localized or generalized hard skin, but excludes hyperkeratoses. Some of these conditions are distinct, primary disease entities, some are part of other diseases, such as systemic lupus erythematosus, and a few are iatrogenic.

Those considered here include localized scleroderma, better known as morphoea. This may occur in single or multiple discs or plaques, configurations such as linear or *en coup de sabre* or, to make matters difficult, in a rare generalized form which may affect the whole trunk or limbs, but without systemic effects. Morphoea may be superficial and of only cosmetic significance, but it can also involve deeper tissues, causing severe deformities of the face and limbs with limitation of respiration or locomotion.

Systemic sclerosis typically involves the extremities with Raynaud's phenomenon, sclerosis of the skin, telangiectasia and calcinosis. A variety of pulmonary, gastrointestinal, renal and other systemic symptoms and characteristic antibody patterns are also present. In typical presentation the condition is easily diagnosed, but when seen early or in atypical form, it can be a challenge to the most experienced dermatologist. The writer does not feel that CRST and CREST (calcinosis, Raynaud's phenomenon, oesophageal involvement, sclerosis, telangiectasia) syndromes are distinct entities. Lichen sclerosus et atrophicus is distinct, and is normally easily diagnosed by dermatologists (or less often by gynaecologists) in its full-blown form, but not so easily when seen, for example, in children without perineal involvement; such cases may need a good quality biopsy to distinguish them from morphoea. One also sees examples of mixed connective tissue disease which defy classification, in spite of modern immunological aids.

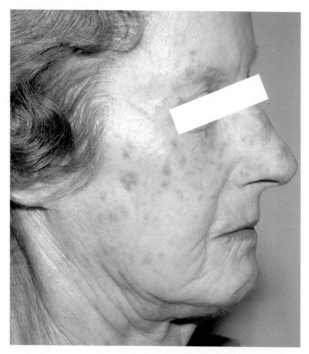

Fig. 10 The characteristic facies of systemic sclerosis. There are vertical furrows around the mouth and a pinched expression, together with a few telangiectases.

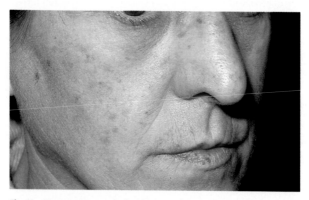

Fig. 11 More pronounced telangiectases, characteristic of CRST syndrome.

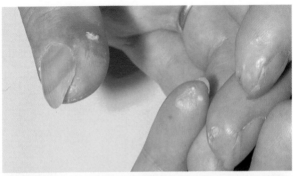

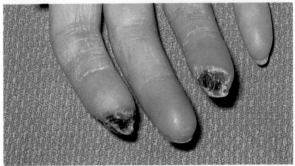

Fig. 12 Some of the changes seen in the fingers in CRST syndrome include smooth, waxy swelling and discharge of calcium (upper) and necrosis of the fingertips (lower).

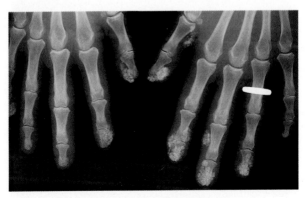

Fig. 13 An X-ray of calcinotic fingers in CRST syndrome.

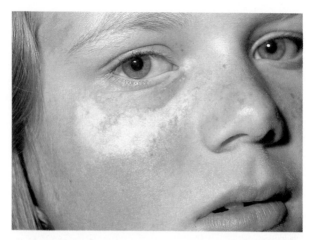

Fig. 14 A plaque of morphoea on the face which, although unsightly, is not harmful and may resolve into paper-thin skin. Extensive involvement of the face, often of segmental distribution, may be associated with hemiatrophy and other deformities.

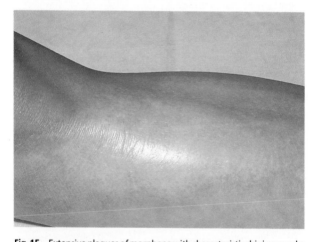

Fig. 15 Extensive plaques of morphoea with characteristic shininess and a yellow, waxy appearance. In early and active cases there is often an advancing erythematous edge and sometimes multiple small raindrop-like lesions of morphoea are present. Very rarely, it is generalized and can encase whole limbs or much of the body in an armour-like carapace, which can interfere with respiration and limb movement and cause severe deformity.

Lichen sclerosus et atrophicus

This condition commonly affects the vulva in adult women and sometimes in children. In children, sexual abuse must be excluded, especially if the lesions are haemorrhagic. When it involves only the vulva, particularly in elderly women, diagnosis can be difficult both clinically and histologically. Frequently, however, the diagnosis is made obvious by examination of the perianal skin. A full examination will often reveal lesions elsewhere, either plaques, or sometimes groups of white spots.

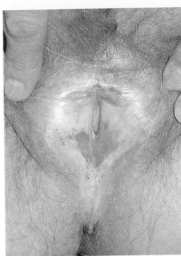

Fig. 16 Lichen sclerosus et atrophicus of the vulva (left). Examination of the perianal skin (lower) often helps to confirm the diagnosis.

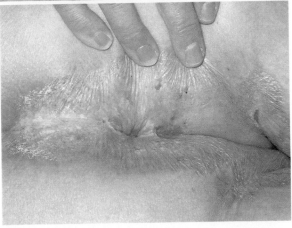

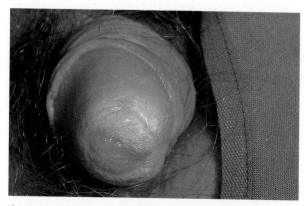

Fig. 17 The effect of lichen sclerosus on the penis, sometimes called balanitis xerotica obliterans. It can affect the glans penis and cause stenosis of the meatal orifice or the prepuce.

Dermatomyositis

Although both neurologists and rheumatologists may consider polymyositis to be quite common, a full-blown picture of dermatomyositis is only occasionally seen by dermatologists. Early diagnosis, before any significant muscular weakness has developed, should not prove difficult for the experienced dermatologist, as appearances are characteristic. Prompt clinical diagnosis is important because confirmation by muscle biopsy and biochemical tests is not always straightforward. Many of the patients whom dermatologists see with this condition have an internal neoplasm.

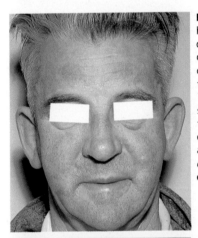

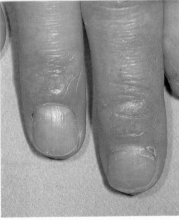

Fig. 18 The face and hands of a patient with dermatomyositis showing characteristic involvement of the forehead and the fingers.
The patient had only slight muscle weakness at this stage, but did have difficulty in swallowing and was shown to have carcinoma of the oesophagus.

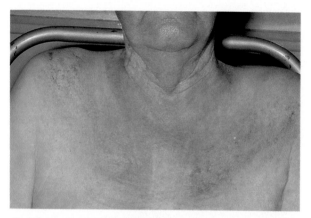

Fig. 19 An extensive eruption of dermatomyositis on the chest.

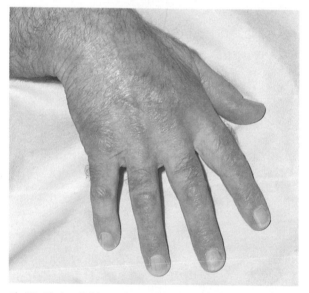

Fig. 20 The hand of the previous patient, who was at this stage moribund with carcinoma of the bronchus.

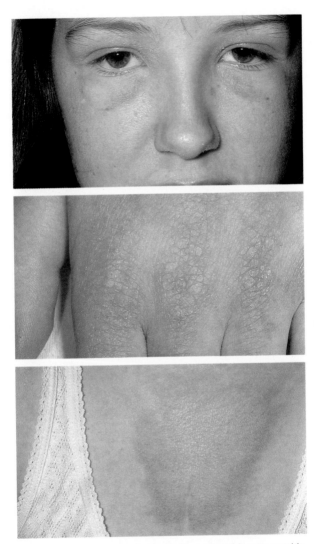

Fig. 21 A child who presented with a florid eruption of dermatomyositis (which was easily diagnosed clinically), together with the rapid development of severe muscle weakness. The latter was effectively controlled with systemic steroids. Despite the continuation of the course for several years, the patient has been fortunate in not developing any unpleasant complications, such as muscle wasting or calcinosis, although skin changes are still present.

In some cases of systemic lupus erythematosus and dermatomyositis, early diagnosis and active therapeutic intervention can be life-saving. In most of the other conditions in this group, however, overactive treatment can be life-threatening rather than helpful and proper management can tax the skill of the dermatologist to the utmost. Fortunately, it does seem possible that, with the further development of specific antibodies, the diagnosis of these illnesses will become much less difficult.

Metabolic and Endocrine Disorders

Many metabolic and endocrine disorders affect the skin, and the dermatological manifestations are often the first to appear.

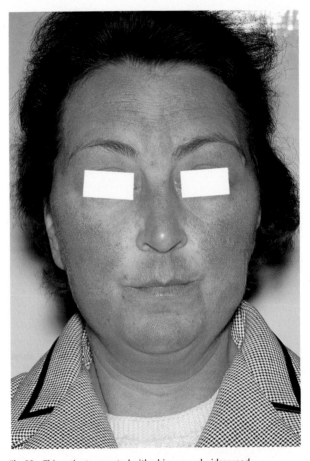

Fig. 22 This patient presented with a bizarre and widespread *Trichophyton rubrum* infection with nail involvement. A history of psychiatric disturbance, together with facial mooning, abdominal striae and hypertension indicated Cushing's syndrome. Partial ablation of the suprarenal glands cured the psychiatric problems and caused a marked decrease in facial mooning.

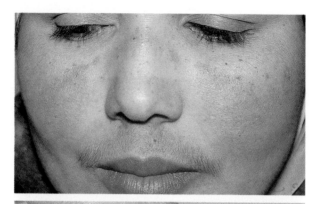

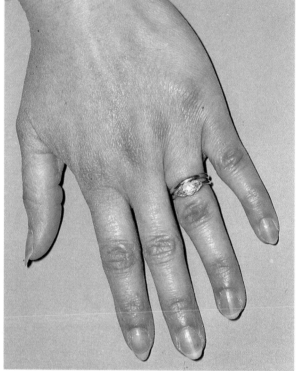

Fig. 23 Addison's disease (suprarenal deficiency). This patient presented with mild facial pigmentation and facial mooning (upper), the result of prolonged cortisone treatment. Mild pigmentation of the hands was also evident (lower). This condition often appears in a much more striking form.

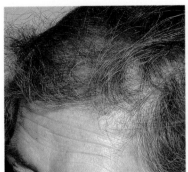

Fig. 24 Hypothyroidism. This condition is characterized by coarse features and thinning hair. Although quite obvious in this case, thyroid disorders are often difficult to diagnose clinically.

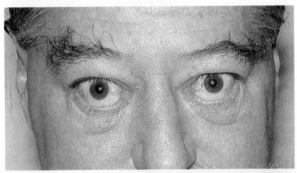

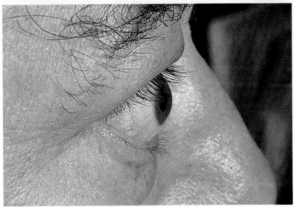

Fig. 25 Hyperthyroidism. Despite a thyroidectomy several years previously, which controlled most of the symptoms (such as tachycardia, nervousness and weight loss), as well as returning the T4 level to normal, this patient presented with severe persisting exophthalmos.

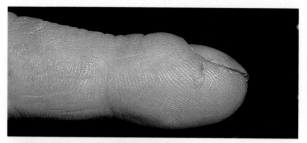

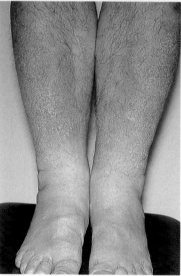

Fig. 26 Acropachy. The same patient exhibiting acrophachy (upper), a much rarer manifestation of thyroid disease which resembles, but is distinct from, finger clubbing. Pretibial myoedema (left) was also evident. The recommended treatments had no effect and the condition resolved spontaneously within several years.

Xanthomatosis

The name xanthomata indicates the common yellow colour of the lesions, but they may also be skin-coloured or white. They can be localized or widespread in distribution, and there are many descriptive terms (disseminated, localized, tuberous, tendinous, plane, xanthelasma palpebrarum) used to describe variations in appearance of the lesions. Their association with systemic conditions such as diabetes mellitus and heart disease, and their familial occurrence have long been recognized. When it became easy to measure lipoproteins, cholesterol and triglycerides, some biochemical order was introduced, especially with Frederickson's classification. Standard textbooks now offer tables which link xanthoma patterns with different types of hyperlipidaemia, but such tables often oversimplify this difficult subject.

Some xanthomata, especially the disseminated plane ones, may indicate a gammopathy. Pseudoxanthoma elasticum is a separate, rare entity. Xanthelasma palpebrarum is commonly no more than a cosmetic disability.

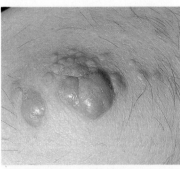

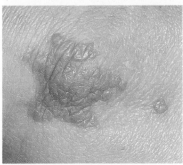

Fig. 27 Xanthomata. The lesions may appear as nodules (upper) or plaques (lower), especially on the elbows.

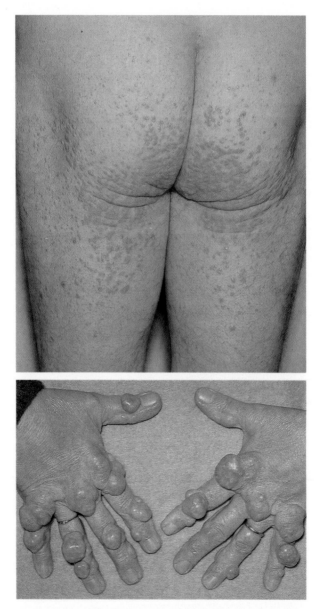

Fig. 28 Widespread, disseminated eruptions of xanthomata appearing as both small and gross lesions.

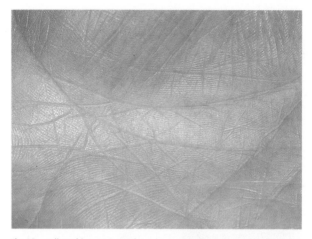

Fig. 29 Yellow skin creases on the palms may be found in association with some cases of xanthomatosis.

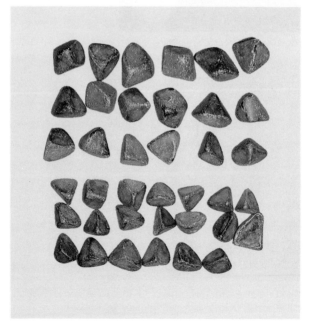

Fig. 30 Gallstones removed from a patient who presented with xanthomata and then rapidly developed billiary colic.

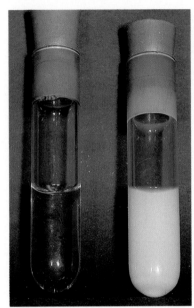

Fig. 31 Milky serum (right) is characteristic of hyperlipidaemia, various types of which may be associated with xanthomatosis.

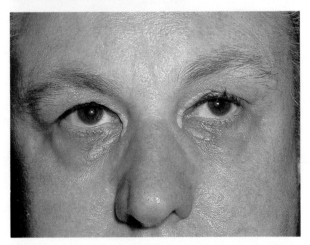

Fig. 32 Xanthelasmata of the eyelids. This is usually an isolated condition, but all cases should be investigated to exclude hyperlipidaemia.

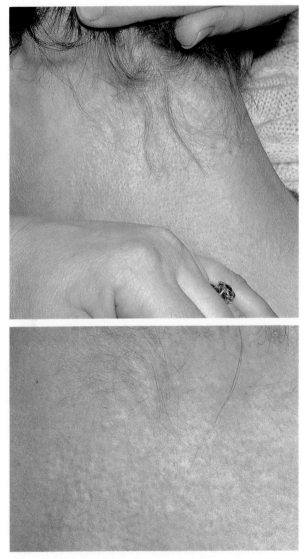

Fig. 33 Lesions of pseudoxanthoma elasticum. This is an uncommon condition, of which there are several types. It may be associated with changes in the blood vessels, for example in the retina, where angioid streaks may be seen. It may also be a cause of significant or lethal haemorrhage, for example from the stomach.

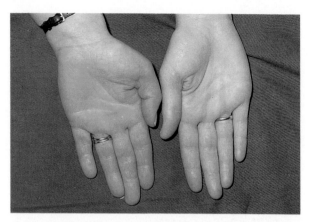

Fig. 34 The palm of a patient with hypercarotinaemia (left) compared with a normal palm. This yellow pigmentation is uncommon. It may be seen in food faddists who consume large amounts of carotene-containing foods and in children who overindulge in satsumas, but has also been recognized in patients with apparently normal diets. It is easily distinguished from jaundice since the conjunctivae are not coloured in hypercarotinaemic patients.

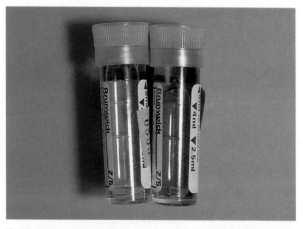

Fig. 35 Normal serum (left) compared with what could be carotinaemic serum. The colour of the latter was, in fact, due to a proprietary preparation containing canthaxanthene, which the patient had been using to obtain an artificial suntan.

Sarcoidosis and the Sarcoid Reaction

This subject continues to fascinate not only dermatologists but also chest physicians, ophthalmologists, orthopaedic surgeons and many others. There is still much to be learned about the causation of sarcoidosis and its investigation and management can be difficult.

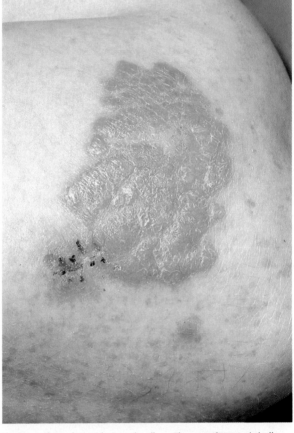

Fig. 36 Lesions of sarcoidosis on the elbow. These are characteristically thickened, well-defined and slightly mauve. The diagnosis was confirmed histologically and although the level of serum angiotensin-converting enzyme was abnormal, detailed investigations showed no other evidence of sarcoidosis. The lesions resolved spontaneously but reappeared after several years, again with no evidence of systemic illness.

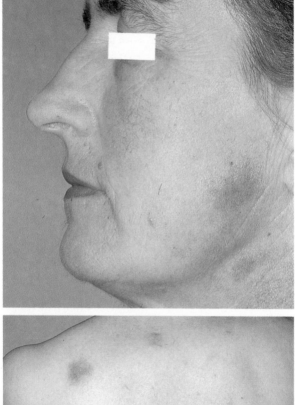

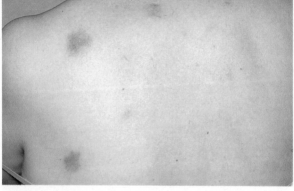

Fig. 37 Widespread sarcoid lesions. These are vascular in appearance and remained unaffected by topical and intralesional steroids. This appearance used to be termed angiolupoid. Several years later, the same patient presented with dactylitis. This disappeared rapidly and completely with hydroxychloroquine administered over 2-3 months. It recurred 2 years later, but was again controlled with hydroxychloroquine treatment.

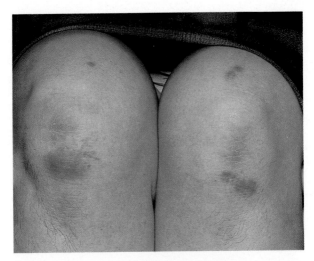

Fig. 38 The knees are a site at which sarcoids often appear.

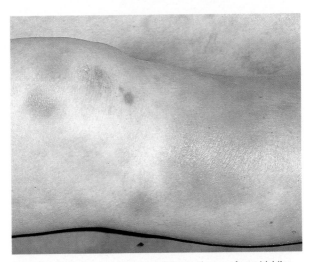

Fig. 39 Sarcoidosis may present as erythema nodosum, often with hilar gland enlargement in the chest. In this unusual case, large red plaques of erythema nodosum are present but among these is a small mauve lesion. Biopsy showed the former to be erythema nodosum and the latter a small sarcoid.

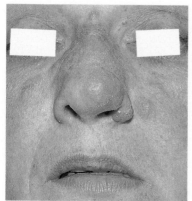

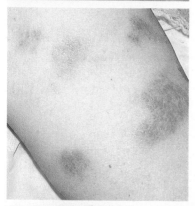

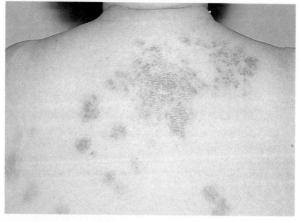

Fig. 40 Widespread sarcoid lesions involving the face, leg and back. In this case, not only were the superficial tissues of the nose involved, but also the nasal mucosa, causing severe obstruction.

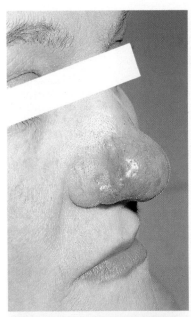

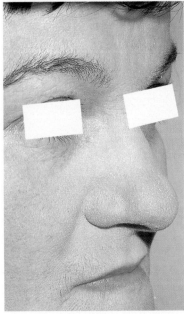

Fig. 41 Sarcoid lesions on the nose (upper). These could be concealed (lower) using covering makeup.

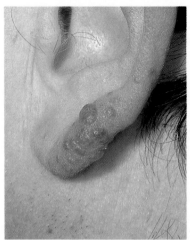

Fig. 42 This case of sarcoidosis arose spontaneously in the ear. There was no history of trauma, such as ear-piercing, to account for it. It was initially thought to be an angioma, but the lesion was much too solid. The diagnosis of sarcoidosis was confirmed histologically.

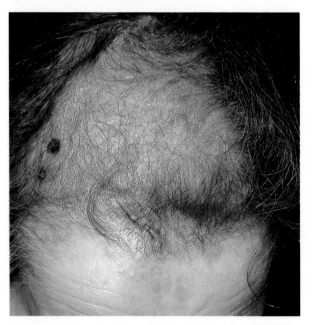

Fig. 43 Atrophic scarring lesions with alopecia in the scalp, and lesions on the forehead.

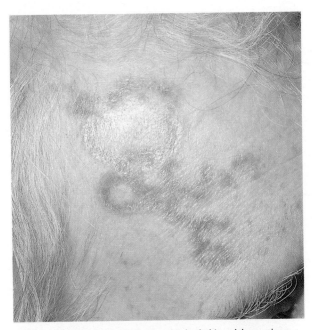

Fig. 44 Annular lesions on the forehead. In both this and the previous case, the histology suggested sarcoid. However, not all such cases represent sarcoidosis or the sarcoid reaction in the true sense. Some of them may be granuloma annulare, Miescher's granuloma, or necrobiosis.

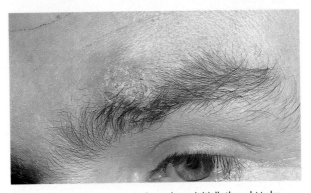

Fig. 45 A localized scaly lesion in the eyebrow, initially thought to be warty tuberculosis. Histological examination showed tuberculoid granuloma with some caseation, but no other signs of tuberculosis were evident and the tuberculin test was negative.

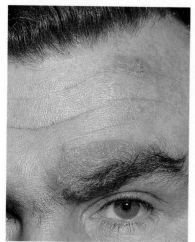

Fig. 46 After 6 months the lesion had spread considerably and it was thought that atypical myocobacteria might be responsible. The patient kept boa constrictors (imported from South America, where they are subject to tuberculosis). Radiological examination of the serpents was negative, and no mycobacteria were identified in their faeces.

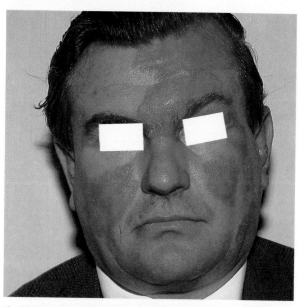

Fig. 47 The same patient 3 years later showing widespread manifest sarcoidosis, which had grown worse during treatment with antituberculous chemotherapy and systemic steroids. All lesions showed a typical sarcoid histology with a negative tuberculin test and a positive Kveim test.

Lymphocytes and the Skin

There are few dermatological conditions in which lymphocytes do not play a part. They may appear in large numbers in conditions as diverse as allergic contact dermatitis, lichen planus and malignant melanoma. There are also numerous clinically nondescript conditions in which lymphocytes collect around the blood vessels in the skin. One does, however, see conditions which can, to some extent, be classified clinically and in which lymphocytes of various classes predominate and play a major part. These may be localized or generalized, benign, harmless and transient, or progressive and lethal. In recent years, much light has been thrown on these conditions by the use of electron microscopy to study the minute details of the nuclei of lymphocytes, and by the use of monoclonal antibodies and other techniques to distinguish the various classes of T and B lymphocytes and their subdivisions.

The classic T cell lymphoma seen by the dermatologist is mycosis fungoides, which is infinitely variable in its presentation. It may start with generalized itching but no other signs, or it may resemble seborrhoeic dermatitis, or even urticaria. It can progress slowly or rapidly in a few years, or, rarely, over 10 or 20 years, and eventually end with fatal multiple fungating tumours. Mycosis fungoides should be suspected when itching is remorseless and uncontrolled by simple remedies, and when lesions are of bizarre defined geometrical shapes, or are infiltrated. Diagnosis in the early stages may be extremely difficult and one may have to perform a dozen or more biopsies in order to make a positive identification.

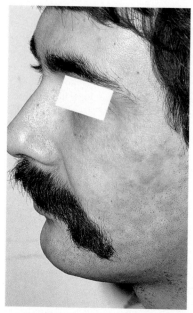

Fig. 48 Lymphocytosis of Jessner, a relatively benign condition, which has recently been shown to be associated with *Borrelia burgdorferi* (Lyme disease).

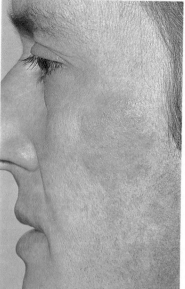

Fig. 49 Non-specific lymphocytosis often appears on exposed areas and resembles discoid lupus erythematosus. Many of these conditions are transitory or recurrent and may respond to antimalarial drugs.

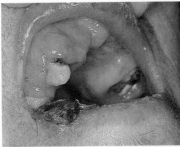

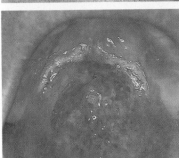

Fig. 50 Leukaemia may present to the dermatologist as oral lesions, as in these cases. Both were initially thought to be pyogenic by the patients' general practitioners, but did not respond to antibiotic treatment. The clinical diagnosis of leukaemia was confirmed haematologically.

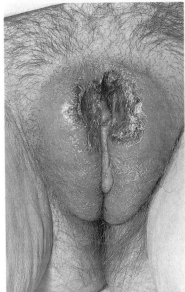

Fig. 51 Acute myeloblastic leukaemia presenting as a vulval ulcer.

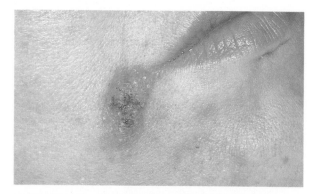

Fig. 52 This patient presented with a hyperkeratotic and scaly area adjoining the angle of the mouth. It was referred as a wart but biopsy, haematological examination and the presence of an enlarged spleen and lymph nodes suggested leukaemia. The patient died 3 days later.

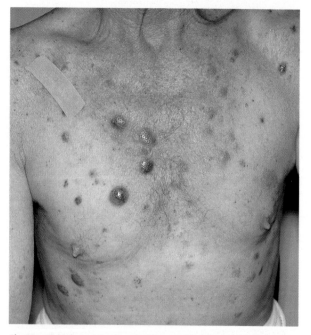

Fig. 53 Multiple nodular deposits of generalized distribution. Previously termed lymphosarcoma, such conditions can now be more adequately classified, usually as B cell lymphomas.

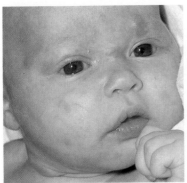

Fig. 54 Similar lesions to those shown in Fig. 53 may occur in young babies, presenting considerable problems in diagnosis and management.

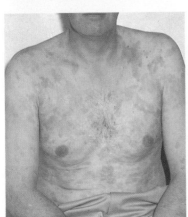

Fig. 55 Mycosis fungoides. This case responded initially to treatment with electronbeam therapy but after 4 years (lower) the condition had become worse.

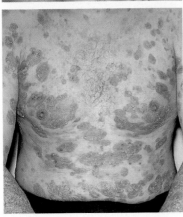

Fig. 56 The same patient a further 4 years later, showing how closely mycosis fungoides can resemble psoriasis.

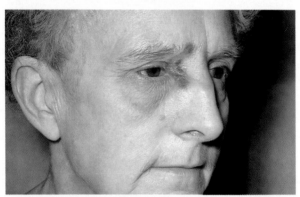

Fig. 57 Mycosis fungoides at an early stage, showing a close resemblance to seborrhoeic dermatitis.

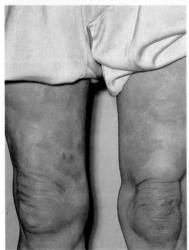

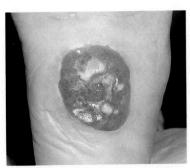

Fig. 58 The same patient 1 year later showing a fungating tumour on the sole. Death occurred 3 years later due to multiple fungating tumours.

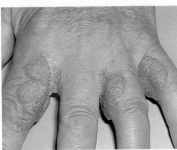

Fig. 59 Mycosis fungoides. This established case shows how variable the condition may be.

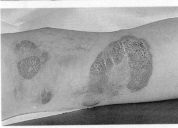

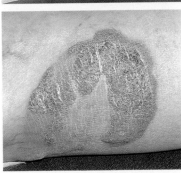

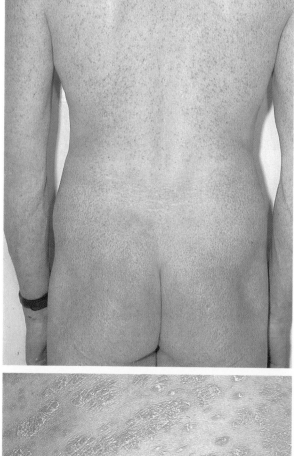

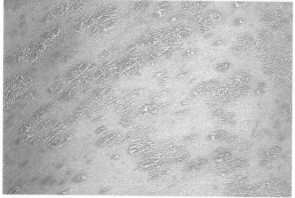

Fig. 60 Poikiloderma. This condition may be an early indication of lymphoma. Sometimes, however, it is benign and remains so, as in this case.

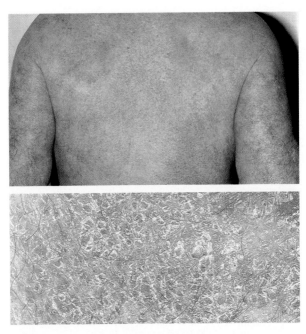

Fig. 61 In some cases poikiloderma may be generalized and associated with intolerable itching, yet may not manifest as frank lymphoma for many years.

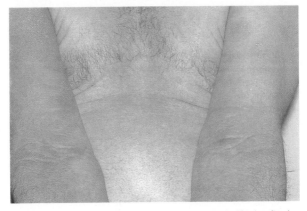

Fig. 62 Sézary syndrome. This may present with urticaria-like, but fixed, lesions.

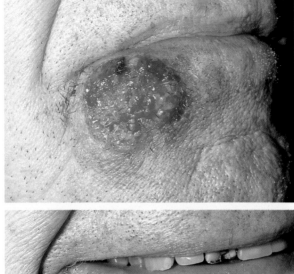

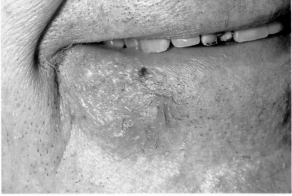

Fig. 63 This patient presented with an acute peculiar granuloma-like lesion (upper) following an insect bite. After 1 week of simple antibiotic treatment (lower) it had resolved almost completely. Histological and haematological examination indicated chronic lymphatic leukaemia, which responded to treatment.

Dermatitis Artefacta

Dermatitis artefacta is an eruption produced by self-inflicted trauma. It must not be confused with other conditions, such as lichen simplex, which are artificial in the sense that they are produced by rubbing or scratching the skin, since these are usually due to an underlying pruritus. Deliberate self-damage for purposes of malingering and gaining compensation is also outside the definition of dermatitis artefacta, since the former is not usually associated with psychiatric illness. Patients with dermatitis artefacta may be described as having 'hysterical personalities' and will deny that the lesions are produced artificially, even when confronted with this suggestion. Those with a medical background will often employ ingenious methods to produce artificial lesions, even to the extent of injecting themselves with bacterial cultures; others may use techniques such as scratching, rubbing or applying caustic chemicals to the skin.

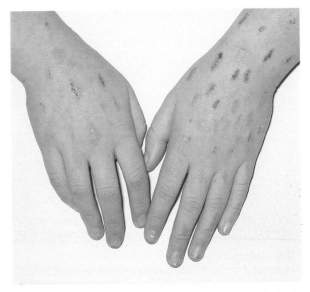

Fig. 64 Dermatitis artefacta. These bilateral linear lesions on the backs of the hands were self-inflicted because of a school phobia.

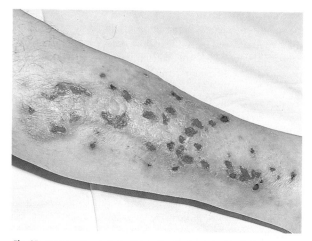

Fig. 65 Dermatitis artefacta. This patient insisted that the lesions were due to industrial dermatitis. They persisted when occlusive bandages were applied to the leg. When a sheet of polythene was placed under the dressing without the patient's knowledge, it was found to be perforated with innumerable needle pricks on removal. This case was certainly on the borderline between dermatitis artefacta and malingering, but the patient did have hysterical manifestations, including aphonia.

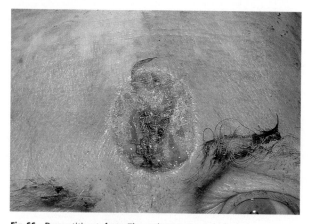

Fig. 66 Dermatitis artefacta. The patient strenuously denied any knowledge of how this lesion might have arisen. A biopsy of the lesion in its early stages (left) was reported as showing changes consistent with mycosis fungoides. When observed without his knowledge, it was found that the patient was using a small set of pocket tools to probe the skin. The

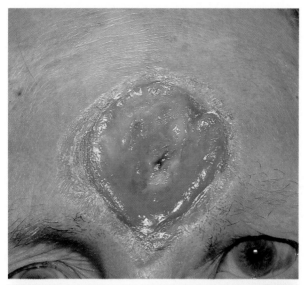

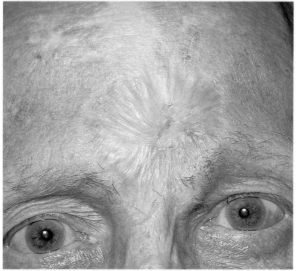

self-inflicted damage was so extreme that the lesion penetrated the frontal sinus (upper). Application of an occlusive dressing allowed the lesion to heal completely after 2 months (lower) but it recurred soon after the dressing was removed. Psychiatric opinion stated that there was no emotional disturbance involved.

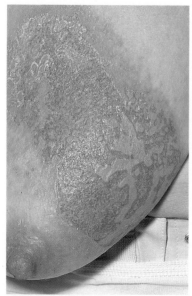

Fig. 67 Dermatitis artefacta. This patient constantly suggested that the unnatural looking erosion on her breast was due to cancer, a belief supported by both her family and general practitioner. Several biopsies revealed no carcinomatous changes.

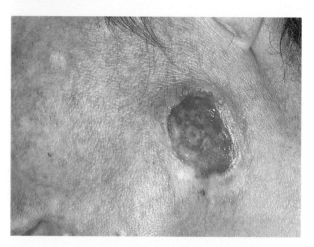

Fig. 68 Dermatitis artefacta. This facial lesion is not unlike a rodent ulcer and the patient was convinced that she had cancer. She worked in a hospital and had, amongst other things, hysterical backache for which she was trying to claim compensation. It was not discovered how she produced the lesion but it continued to reappear, even after excision and skin grafting on several occasions.

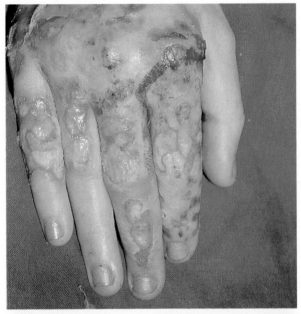

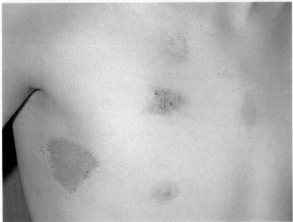

Fig. 69 Eruptions of dermatitis artefacta are often of unusual appearance and distribution. This dermatitis of the hand (upper) looks grossly unnatural and was produced artificially, as were the odd-looking patches on the chest (lower) of a separate patient.

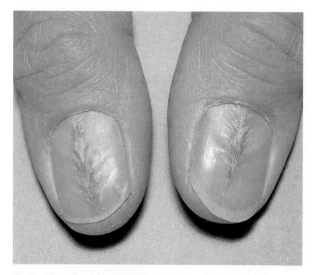

Fig. 70 Linear furrows of the thumbnails. These were produced by continual picking at the proximal nailfold.

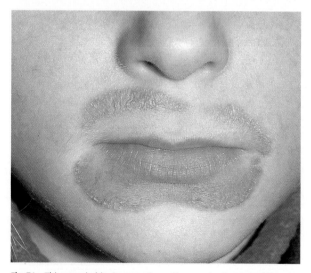

Fig. 71 This remarkable circumoral eruption was due to constant lip licking. Although the patient was observed to continually lick her lips throughout the consultation, both she and her mother strenuously denied that she ever did such a thing.

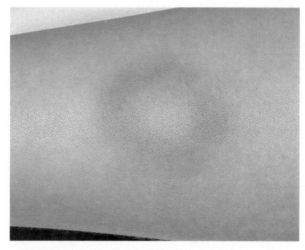

Fig. 72 A suction blister on the forearm.

Miscellaneous Conditions

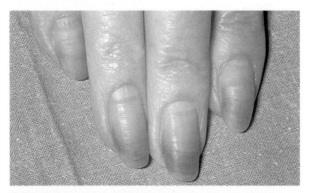

Fig. 73 Yellow nail syndrome is an indication of lymphoedema. This patient had bilateral lymphoedema of the legs and pleural effusions. Her nails had been fruitlessly treated with topical systemic fungicides over a long period of time.

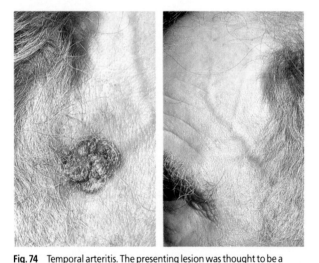

Fig. 74 Temporal arteritis. The presenting lesion was thought to be a malignant melanoma. It was, in fact, a pigmented basal cell carcinoma (left) which was curetted and cauterized. On injection of a local anaesthetic with adrenalin, the patient remarked that his headache was cured. The underlying temporal artery was thick and tortuous, as was the contralateral vessel (right). The blood sedimentation rate was 80mm in an hour, falling to 18mm after a week of treatment with systemic steroids.

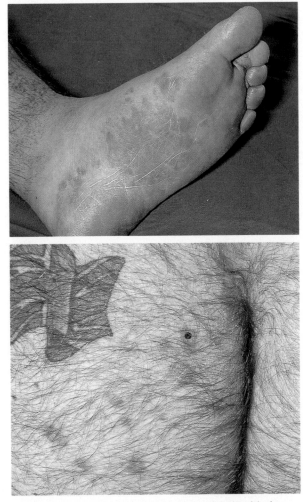

Fig. 75 AIDS. This patient had purplish plaques on the soles of the feet and on the lower legs, and infiltrated papules on the thighs and buttocks. He was a promiscuous homosexual who had been visiting the United States. All of the lesions showed the histology of Kaposi's sarcoma, which was also affecting the patient's bowel. He survived for some 6 months.

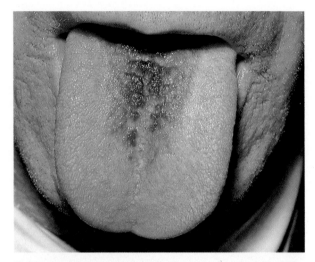

Fig. 76 This patient has a black, hairy tongue. Many people are happy to live with this condition, but others find it quite distressing. Recommended treatment, such as scraping with the edge of a glass slide, is seldom of lasting effect.

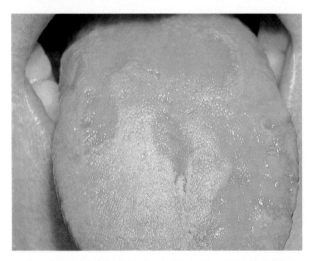

Fig. 77 Geographical tongue. This condition is characterized by transitory migratory plaques on the dorsum of the tongue. Many patients are unaware of this, but others become totally obsessed. It is quite benign but does not respond to treatment.

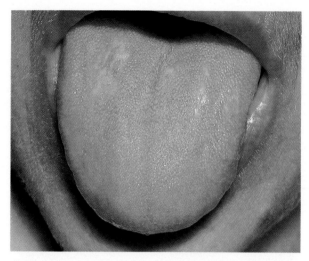

Fig. 78 These small, whitish areas on the tongue were caused by sucking very strong peppermints, but disappeared when the patient gave up this practice. The condition had previously been regarded as premalignant leukoplakia.

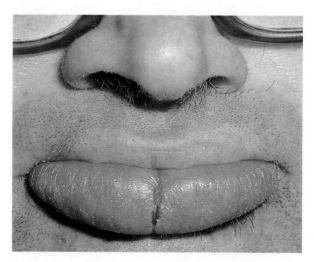

Fig. 79 Granulomatous cheilitis. The lower lip of this patient was thick, fissured and deformed. Histology showed sarcoid-like granulomas, but no other signs of sarcoidosis were evident. Plastic surgery improved the condition considerably.

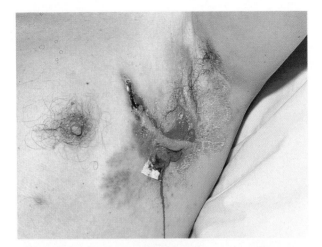

Fig. 80 Hidradenitis suppurativa. The axillae show discharging sinuses and fibrous and keloidal scars. The condition resolved completely with prolonged tetracycline therapy, but more severe cases may require wide surgical excision of the entire axillary skin.

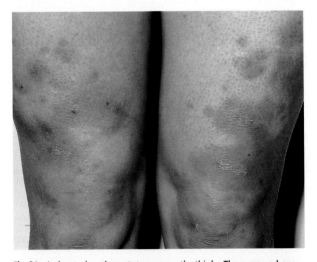

Fig. 81 Indurated erythematous areas on the thighs. These can perhaps be regarded as an exaggerated type of chilblain. The condition has been termed 'equestrian cold panniculitis' because it has been described in those who ride horses in cold weather wearing unsuitable clothing, such as thin, tight jeans.

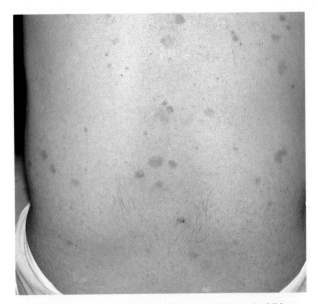

Fig. 82 Pityriasis lichenoides chronica. This commonly occurs in children, but may be seen at any age. It causes small, pleomorphic, itchy papules and crusted lesions which may persist for long periods. It may be misdiagnosed as repeated attacks of chickenpox or confused with insect bites.

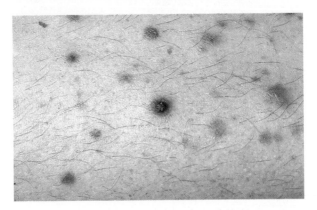

Fig. 83 Pityriasis lichenoides et varioliformis acuta. The lesions are more angry and pustular than those of pityriasis lichenoides chronica and show the histology of vasculitis.

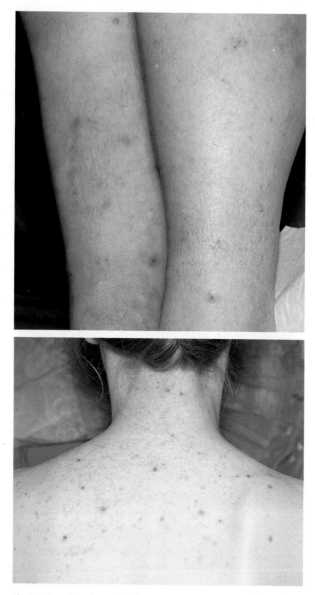

Fig. 84 Eruptions due to bites from cat fleas (upper) or infestation with headlice (lower) may be confused with pityriasis lichenoides.

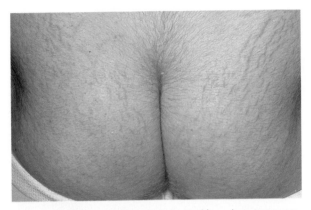

Fig. 85 Purple striae on the buttocks. Striae gravidarum in pregnancy are well recognized but striae distensae in non-pregnant women, or in men, may cause confusion. In this case they were due to Cushing's syndrome, a very rare cause.

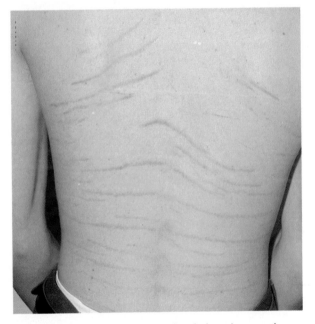

Fig. 86 Multiple striae. It is by no means the rule that striae appear in young people due to sudden weight loss or gain; they often arise for no apparent reason. They may cause concern, but usually fade spontaneously.

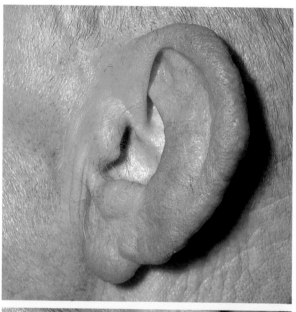

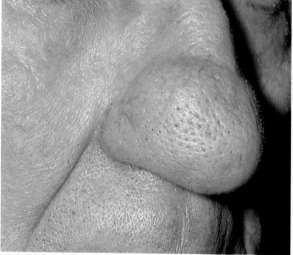

Fig. 87 Relapsing polychondritis. This rare, but striking, condition most commonly presents as recurrent painful erythema and swelling of one or both ears (upper). It can also affect other cartilages, such as the nose (lower), costochondral cartilage and even the larynx.

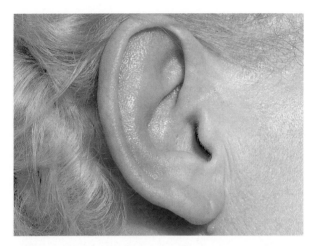

Fig. 88 Polychondritis affecting the ear. Minor manifestations of this are probably not uncommon, but the fully developed polychondritis is very rare and may ultimately lead to considerable deformity of the ear. The condition may be mistaken for erysipelas.

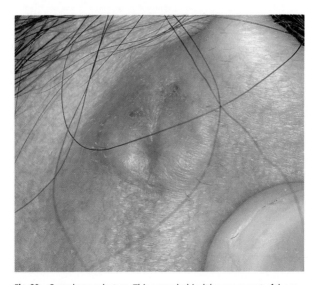

Fig. 89 Granuloma sulcatum. This occurs behind the upper part of the ear in spectacle wearers and can be extremely persistent. This patient had contact lenses fitted and had the lesion excised 3 times, with a recurrence each time. On no occasion was there histological evidence of malignancy.

Granuloma annulare

This condition is typically seen in children and young adults. When it occurs for the first time in adults, especially if widespread or atypical, one should consider the presence of diabetes mellitus. It should be emphasized however, that most patients with granuloma annulare do not have diabetes mellitus and do not develop it. The lesions tend to develop on the distal portions of the extremities, although the condition may be generalized. Even when characteristic, it is often mistaken for fungal infection and some patients may undergo treatment with systemic antifungal drugs, even toxic ones such as ketoconazole. Occasionally, the lesions will disappear if traumatized, for example by freezing or injection of a local anaesthetic. More commonly, however, they persist as a cosmetic nuisance and eventually resolve spontaneously. Atypical cases may be confusing and it can be difficult to distinguish between granuloma annulare, annular sarcoid of the scalp and other rarer forms of granuloma.

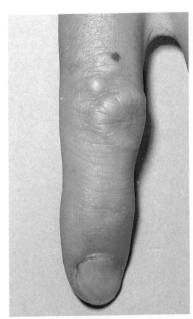

Fig. 90 Granuloma annulare. The lesions most often arise over bony prominences, particularly on the knuckles and finger joints.

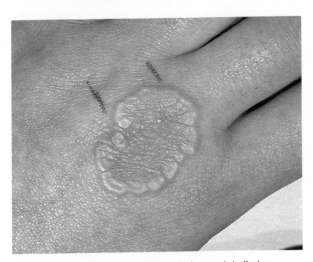

Fig. 91 This lesion of granuloma annulare is characteristically ring-shaped, with a distinct edge consisting of bead-like papules. The edge may occasionally consist of a continuous band, but is usually comprised of discrete elements.

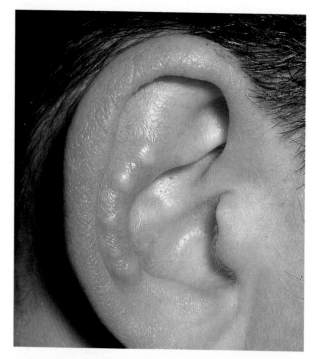

Fig. 92 Granuloma annulare may occur on the ear (as in this case) or, more commonly, on the feet.

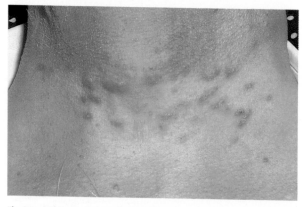

Fig. 93 Atypical lesions on the neck of an elderly diabetic patient which were histologically characteristic of granuloma annulare.

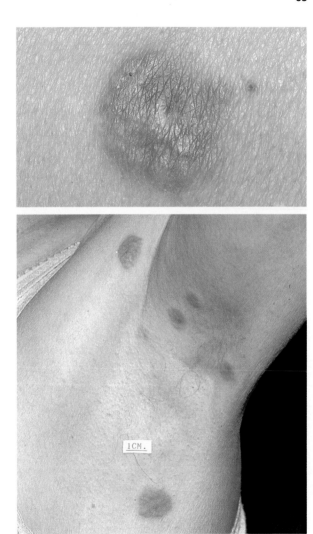

Fig. 94 This patient presented with a single lesion on the left flank (upper). It was extremely hard and suggested a secondary malignant deposit or an atypical basal cell carcinoma. Biopsy showed typical granuloma annulare histology, and when seen 1 month later (lower), the patient had developed multiple lesions. One lesion was injected with triamcinolone acetonide suspension, after which it flattened satisfactorily. However, those lesions which were not injected disappeared equally rapidly.

Necrobiosis lipoidica diabeticorum

Necrobiosis occurs in both adults and children and is commonly, but not invariably, associated with diabetes. Some children may present with lesions of necrobiosis as the first manifestation of diabetes; other cases may develop when diabetes is already manifest.

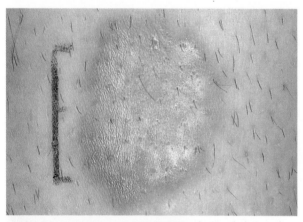

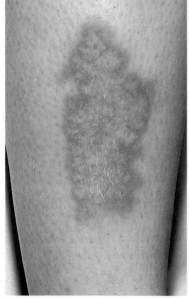

Fig. 95 The lesions of necrobiosis occur most frequently on the anterior shins and may be unilateral, as seen here, or bilateral.

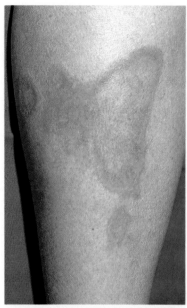

Fig. 96 The lesions are characteristically circumscribed, yellowish, waxy and shiny, with telangiectasia and sometimes atrophy.

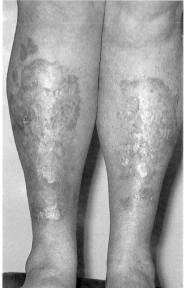

Fig. 97 Bilateral lesions in a case of necrobiosis which persisted for 30 years. The lesions frequently broke down and ulcerated, always responding to supporting bandages. The condition eventually resolved spontaneously. Some years later, fulminating pyoderma gangrenosum developed in the same site and proved fatal.

Disorders of the Scalp and Hair

Unfortunately, scalp disorders, apart from ringworm, are not usually amenable to simple curative treatment. Disorders of the scalp and of hair growth, however mild, often produce profound emotional disturbance and many patients may spend large sums on dubious practitioners in the hope of growing hair. Children with hair abnormalities need a very careful and full clinical examination of the skin, teeth, bones and joints; chromatography of the urine for abnormal amino acids should also form part of the investigation. Some of these conditions are significant, in that they are associated with multiple defects, including mental abnormalities.

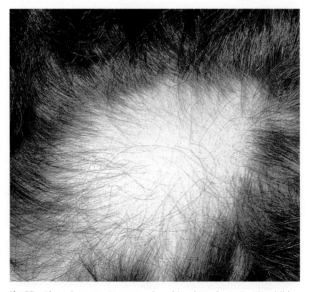

Fig. 98 Alopecia areata. In cases such as this, where the patient is a child with only a single patch of hair loss, the prognosis is good and the hair will probably regrow without treatment.

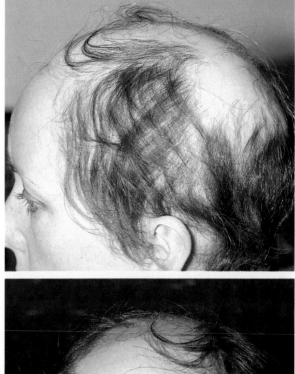

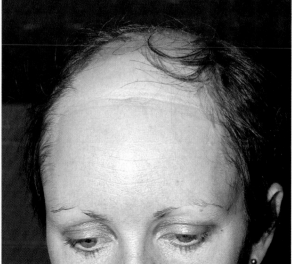

Fig. 99 Alopecia areata. In cases of more extensive hair loss, such as this, the chances of complete and normal regrowth are much smaller. This is also the case when the patient is atopic or when the alopecia is particularly marked around the margins of the scalp (ophiasis).

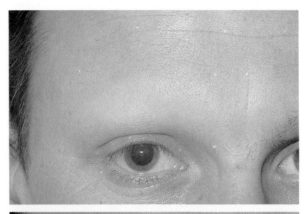

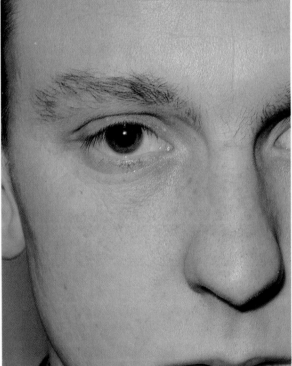

Fig. 100 Alopecia areata of the eyebrows (upper). Local infiltration of the area with triamcinolone caused the hair to regrow satisfactorily (lower), but as soon as the injections were stopped, it fell out again.

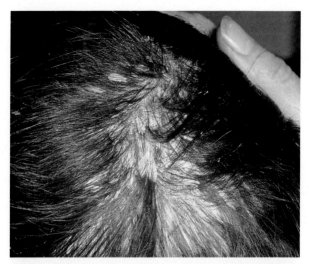

Fig. 101 Seborrhoea capitis. Also known as sheathing pityriasis or *fausse teigne amiantacée*, this condition has a much more alarming appearance than pityriasis capitis, but is easier to treat if the patient will persevere with tar and salicylic acid pomades.

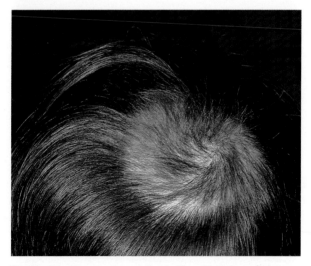

Fig. 102 This appearance is caused by plucking of the hair, producing a partially bald patch with areas of short hair about 1 cm long.

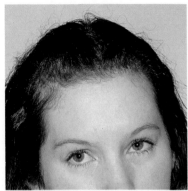

Fig. 103 Traction by certain forms of hairstyle can pull the hair out and cause alopecia, as in this patient who had bilateral temporal alopecia.

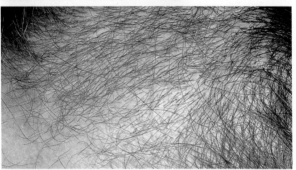

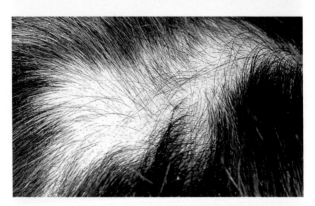

Fig. 104 This bald patch was due to the hair being pulled out during a fight. The dermatologist often sees cases of traumatic alopecia for medicolegal reasons; for example, the scalp may be burnt during the course of a permanent wave, producing scarring alopecia.

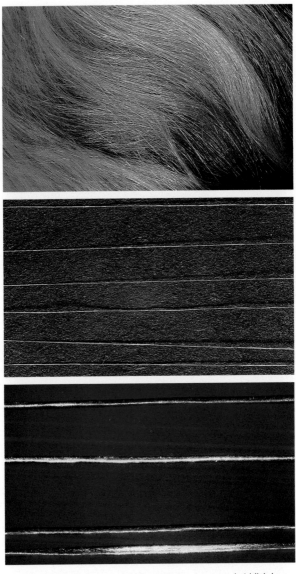

Fig. 105 Brindled hair (upper). Reflected light microscopy (middle) shows twisting of the hairs, as does polarized light (lower). Microscopy slides by courtesy of the Department of Pathology, Kent and Canterbury Hospital.

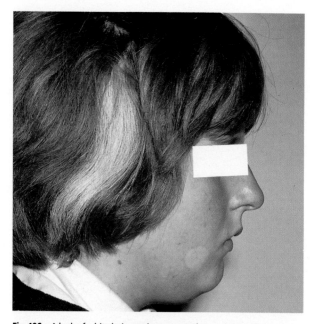

Fig. 106 A lock of white hair may be no more than an interesting abnormality, and in some cases may be considered attractive, but it can be associated with deafness and other abnormalities. It must also be remembered that when new hair grows after alopecia areata, it is often of abnormal texture or colour (commonly white).

Dermatoses Due to Sunlight

The effects of light on the human skin are numerous and complex, so much so that photodermatology is a specialty in its own right. The dermatologist encounters many abnormal reactions to light, varying from temporary and trivial to chronic and disabling, or even life-threatening. The investigation and interpretation of these disorders can be an extreme challenge. It can, for example, be difficult to decide whether sunburn is due to simple overexposure to light, or whether a patient is actually hypersensitive. Abnormal sensitivity to light can manifest itself in infancy and childhood. Congenital porphyria is perhaps the most quoted example of this, although it is actually so rare that few dermatologists ever see a case of it.

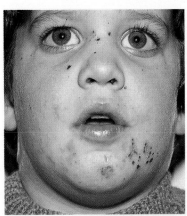

Fig. 107 Congenital porphyria. The child in this case was not, at this stage, greatly inconvenienced by the disease, which can become serious and life-threatening.

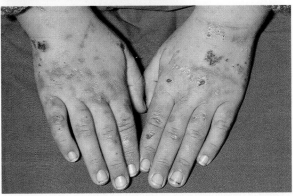

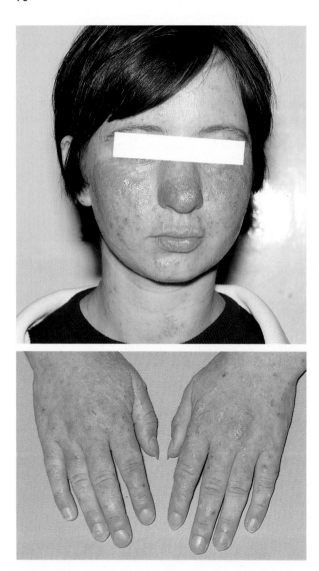

Fig. 108 This patient presented at the age of 3 and remained affected until early adult life. The clinical picture varied from pruriginous papules on exposed areas in early summer to a vesicular form, later adopting an appearance suggestive of atopic eczema. It was variously diagnosed as hydroa aestivale and Hutchinson's summer prurigo, illustrating the difficulty of making a precise diagnosis in these cases.

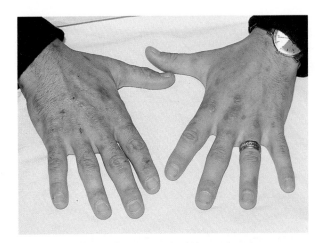

Fig. 109 Hepatic porphyria. This condition may present as only minor blistering of the fingers. It is commonly seen in alcoholics and may be transient. This patient developed symptoms every summer after a holiday in Spain, where it was her habit to consume several bottles of wine a day, but was untroubled once back in England.

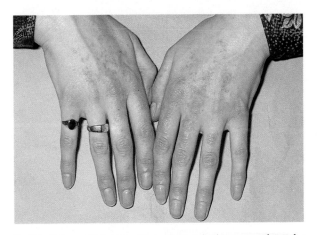

Fig. 110 Polymorphic light eruption on the hands. This common form of light sensitivity can produce various erythematous eruptions, and usually appears on the forearms and face as well as on the hands. Most patients are affected in early spring, but the condition often resolves in late summer. It can be prevented by exposure to UVA in early spring.

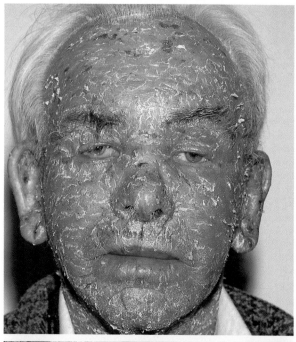
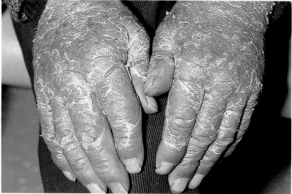

Fig. 111 Exfoliative dermatitis. Light sensitivity can be induced by many drugs and other chemicals. This patient was sensitized by chlorothiazide, given for mild hypertension. He recovered after 3 weeks in hospital, but returned 2 weeks later, having been given bendrofluazide by another doctor.

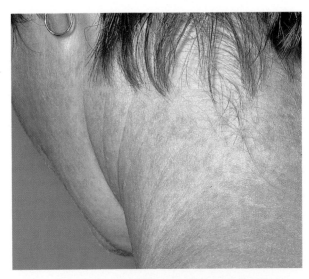

Fig. 112 This patient was sensitized by an antidepressive drug. This type of reaction on exposed areas may be difficult to interpret because it can be mimicked by contact dermatitis due to plants or to aerosol sprays. Note that the areas shaded by the ear and the hair on the neck are spared.

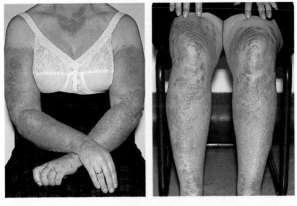

Fig. 113 This patient was sensitized by demethylchlortetracycline. Note the very sharp cut-off on the upper arms (where her sleeves protected her) and the vesicular appearance on the forearms. A similar eruption was present on the legs. This is a highly exaggerated phototoxic sunburn type of reaction. Not all such reactions resolve immediately and permanently once the offending drug is withdrawn.

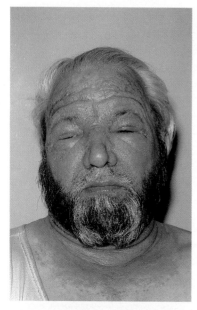

Fig. 114 This patient has become a persistent reactor, to the extent that he is no longer able to leave his house.

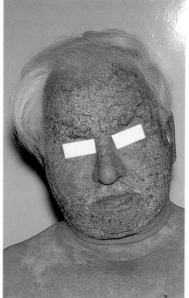

Fig. 115 Some patients develop a reaction so persistent and severe that it simulates lymphoma. The histology is lymphoma-like, with infiltration by atypical mononuclear cells. The condition has been termed actinic reticuloid.

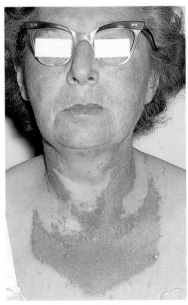

Fig. 116 This light eruption has spared the face but affects the 'v' of the neck. The patient was taking the antimalarial, chloroquine, for rheumatoid arthritis. Antimalarial drugs were once used as oral sunscreening agents, although they are much too dangerous to be employed for this purpose in a routine way. Many topical sunscreening drugs can also act as photosensitizers.

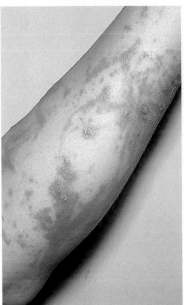

Fig. 117 Many plants can sensitize patients to light. They often produce oddly patterned and streaked eruptions, sometimes with blistering where leaves have brushed against the skin, as in this case.

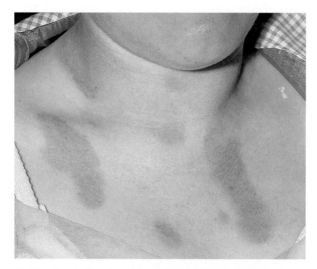

Fig 118 These oddly shaped, brownish patches were due to sensitization by oil of bergamot in perfume.

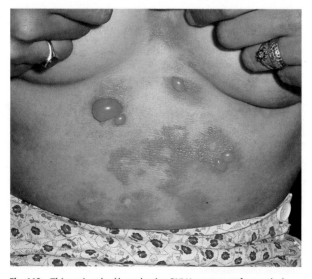

Fig. 119 This patient had been having PUVA treatment for psoriasis but, in spite of the warnings given, she did not cover up adequately when in the sun and the severe bullous eruption which resulted necessitated in-patient hospital treatment.

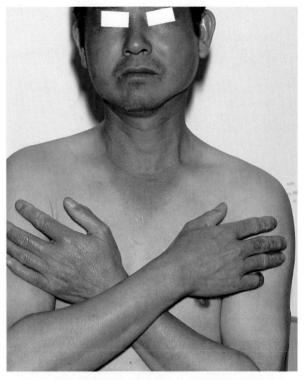

Fig. 120 Industrial sensitization to light. In this case, sensitization was due to cinnamates in a patient who worked in a perfume factory.

INDEX